A Fresh Take on
ERGONOMICS

A Fresh Take on
ERGONOMICS

AVOIDING PAIN IN THE WORKPLACE

Betsy Oldenburg, LMBT, Trager® Practitioner and Tutor

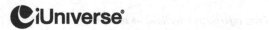

A FRESH TAKE ON ERGONOMICS
AVOIDING PAIN IN THE WORKPLACE

A Fresh Take on Ergonomics, Avoiding Pain in the Workplace
Betsy Oldenburg, LMBT, Trager® Practitioner and tutor

iUniverse books may be ordered through booksellers or by contacting:

iUniverse
1663 Liberty Drive
Bloomington, IN 47403
www.iuniverse.com
1-800-Authors (1-800-288-4677)

ISBN: 978-1-4917-7795-4 (sc)
ISBN: 978-1-4917-7796-1 (e)

Print information available on the last page.

iUniverse rev. date: 10/07/2019

SPECIAL THANKS

Firstly I want to thank my many clients for encouraging me to present and write this material. They were open to listening and implementing these ideas, and verified its value to me. I am immensely grateful to Caitlin Warde for her enthusiasm and early editing, and to Mark Schumacher for finishing the job so willingly. Many thanks to Sara Jane Mann for her diligence in creating clear helpful illustrations and photography. My gratitude to Mars and I Universe for your patience and professionalism. Thank you Connie Pounders for your input, enthusiasm, and dear friendship. I am deeply grateful to Dr. Milton Trager, and my many teachers and colleagues for inspiring me in the field of body/mind awareness. I thank you Lori Loveland for bringing my skills to the medical field, and so much more. And I thank Sky for the nudge to make it mine.

Table of Contents

"We can actually change feelings we have about our own status through the physical positions we take in our bodies."

Amy Cuddy – American social psychologist and Body Language Researcher

INTRODUCTION

Your amazing body was not created to sit for prolonged hours at a desk, hunched over a keyboard. Day after day at the computer, or doing repetitive movements, a body is slowly contorted into a dysfunctional position. Many of us walk around with all manner of aches and pains that we may attribute to a "bad back," or to just getting older, when there is much more involved than we realize. Balance is key.

Whether you are a computer technician, artist, hairdresser, homemaker, teacher or mechanic you can benefit from my knowledge as a Trager® movement re-education practitioner and bodywork therapist for thirty years.

I am compelled to share my experience at the urging of hundreds of my clients who have been helped. They have been able to manage or eliminate their discomfort or pain resulting from extensive computer use, or other jobs that put them in dysfunctional positions.

If you sit at a desk for any length of time, chances are you have thought about, heard about or been given specific advice regarding good ergonomics and better furniture. But I'm here to tell you that there is no perfect chair, or desk, or position that will solve the problem.

My unique experience as a body worker has given me significant insights into how to eliminate the aches and pains that plague many adults in a myriad of professions. This approach differs radically from traditional ergonomic thought and theory. A few of my Helpful Hints were inspired by other sources, but my approach is proven and uniquely my own.

Humans were not meant to sit in a car, and our nervous systems were not designed with the intention of going seventy miles per hour! And frankly, we were not made to sit in one position while holding a book or a tablet, a newspaper, or knitting needles for hours on end. I get a kick out of telling my clients that "chairs are evil!" Truthfully, most people who suffer pain from long periods of time at a desk will heartily agree. **Chairs do not occur in nature,** they are a man-made invention. Our bodies conform to dysfunctional furniture in much of our modern environment. If you are not able to get comfortable in a chair or couch, the problem is not you, rather it is the problem of living with seating that collapses our structure.

New studies are coming out telling us that sitting is as bad for us as smoking. It is being shown that standing on our feet and moving about is what triggers the body to conduct its business of producing the right hormones and other chemical interactions which are vital to life. When we sit, many of those important mechanisms shut down. Other than during our healing sleep time, we are not meant to do any one thing for long stretches of time. We are meant to be moving about in all directions to keep all joints limber and systems functioning.

Our bodies are composed of 65-75% fluid, and soft tissues, or muscles, are meant to be in motion to some extent for most of our waking hours. If I really "tune in" to my body, I cannot sit here writing for more than ten minutes before I need to change my position, or get up to fetch a glass of water, or fold clothes or stretch! (And I love what I'm doing – this is fun! What about the folks who are less enthusiastic about what they are doing?)

Those of us who work at desks, seated, or who work in one position standing or bending, must constantly repress our natural urge to move. We have to damp down our own instincts in order to perform our work, which leads to all sorts of pain. Our physical structure begins breaking down and our minds and hearts do also.

Sitting in meditation or prayer is entirely another matter. When relaxation is our primary aim, we do better. Even so, I would choose to sit in a way that puts my feet as close as possible beneath my center of gravity. More on that later. . .

In an attempt to alleviate the pain brought on by your workplace, you can get a very special expensive ergonomic chair that claims to place you in just "the right" alignment, but my experience has me guess that your relief, if any, will only last for a while. Soon you will feel uncomfortable again, or will hurt as you stand up. You will never find the "right chair." There is no perfect desk set up because we are not made to be in the same situation for extended periods of time day after day.

Poor Posture Being in a position where the head is out forward and chest caving in is called a 'collapsed posture'. Being in this posture too much, can lead to all kinds of health consequences including:

-Neck tension

-Upper back and shoulder pain

-Headaches

-Jaw malfunction and TMJ problems

-Digestive problems and constipation

-Limiting of endorphin hormones, the feel good hormones, leading to irritability and behavioral problems

-Sleep problems, and insomnia

-Anxiety and depression

The Importance of Change!

I urge my clients who sit at a desk all day to *change* chairs mid-morning and mid- afternoon. *Change* the height of your keyboard and screen, *change* the placement of your mouse.

If you are on your feet all day, then change your shoes mid-morning and mid-afternoon.

Even in our sleep, change is best. Did you ever find just the right pillow - the pillow of your dreams? You enjoyed it for a few weeks or months, and then it didn't work anymore? Well it may not be a bad pillow, don't throw it out, just change pillows when one stops working for you. More on pillows in general later.

Notes:

While this book can be helpful for those who are seeking preventative care ideas, it is not meant to replace medical care for substantial, acute and/or chronic issues.

I want to emphasize that my suggestions for stretches and other movement practices here are in no way comprehensive. They are the most basic, general and relevant ones that I share with all of my clients in the limited time we have together. There are certainly volumes available to read regarding stretching and joint care for your particular situation. My main focus is for you to understand the importance of getting your body out of collapse whenever and wherever possible, and to share easy ways to find balance.

Where there are directions for stretching, please do them gently. There is a fine line between a good gentle stretch that gives time for the muscle to lengthen on its own, and overstretching which signals the muscle to guard and is a set up for a painful muscle pull or worse injury. Try to warm up the muscles you are going to stretch with prior movement, or by quickly rubbing them. In general, **tension** is a learned condition of the subconscious mind as taught by The Trager approach® and The Feldenkrais Method which are mentioned later, and it is most beneficial to calm our minds before stretching.

"There is so much to gain from improving your posture. Everybody's interested in the way they look, and then they're astounded to find the other benefits." Janice Novak, Author of Posture, Get It Straight!

FOR YOUR NECK

My Helpful Hint # 1 is **'Zip It Up!'**

The easiest way to find your own most comfortable efficient posture is to pretend zipping up your jacket. I was first exposed to this idea in my training with Dr. Milton Trager.

What do you do when you zip up your jacket? Most likely you hold the front of your jacket at the bottom with one hand and lift your chest slightly, lengthening your torso so that the zipper is straight enough to work smoothly. You can adjust your posture anytime by doing this slight lift of your ribs. Remember to keep your <u>chin level</u> and do not arch your back. Simply focus on elongation of your front, and you will find your head resting in a balanced way on top of your spine, and your shoulders automatically spread back. You may have heard of the idea to imagine a balloon tied to the top of your head. Zipping up is different in that it doesn't require your neck to do the work. **You do not need to exert your back or neck to gain good posture.** Imagine a balloon expanding inside your chest. The 'Zip It Up' can be applied anytime you are sitting, standing, or walking. Zip Up twenty times a day! This tip works even when leaning forward as in riding a bike, or bending over to pick something up. Lead with your chest. Do not pull your head or shoulders back, but consciously lift your sternum, or chest bone. This simple adjustment to your body alignment has a great effect on the whole of your body. It helps your neck to be more comfortable; it makes room in your abdomen for your digestion; it allows for deeper breathing, and it frees up your energy! This way of standing and sitting will give you a look and feel of confidence, grace, power and grounded-ness. Allow your shoulders to hang freely. **Please remember: It should be easy! Good posture should not be hard work!**

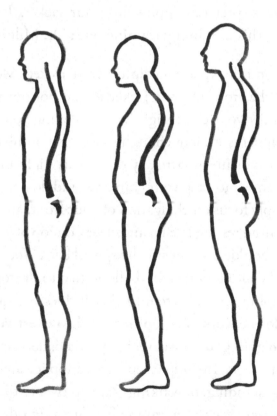

The **'Zip It Up'** is the first tool I teach to help undo the years of your body's forward collapse. You know the slump that happens when you sit in a chair, where your head moves forward, the chest sinks, and the low back rounds. When you collapse forward, or sit on your low back, a cascade of negative consequences ensues. The breath gets shallow and cut off, as does your digestion. It also compresses your internal organs, which can lead to all kinds of pain and disruption. No wonder you hurt! It is the life draining posture we notice in the older person who is bent over, unable to move freely, slowly and sadly acquiescing to gravity.

Another generally good rule of thumb, is when looking down at your keyboard, or up at a plane, look in those directions with your eyes. That way you can leave your head balanced instead of leaning it forward or down. Zip Up your torso and let your eyes do the adjusting. Sometimes you will need to move your head in those directions, but be aware not to overdo it.

Remember your neck is delicate compared to the rest of your spine. Be easy with your neck when possible. It is true that sometimes we need to stretch the front of our neck. I like to say that stars were created so we look up after looking down at all the things we do in a day. In this case lean forward a bit and gently roll your head back, letting it lay on your upper back as you feel a gentle stretch in the front.

"Each of us can develop and more fully realize who we are only when we experience something different and better." Milton Trager, M.D., *Movement As A Way To Agelessness*

SITTING AND CHAIRS

What do you mean I am not supposed to sit in a chair?

Think about where and how you would sit, if there were no chairs. You could sit on the ground with your feet out in front of you, but try it out; how comfortable is that and how long could you last there? You might fold and cross your legs, lean up against a tree, or put some small lift under your tailbone, but for most of us my guess is it wouldn't feel comfortable for long and without collapsing, unless you are a practiced yogini or a two year old. In my experience, the most comfortable seating is on horseback. Of course you could sit on a log, and in that case I would rather straddle the log, than to sit with my feet out in front of me.

Why?

Because anytime your feet are out in front of the body, it invites you to hunch over or collapse the front line of your structure. Our heads are heavy, equivalent in mass to a small bowling ball (eight or ten pounds). Our bodies are designed to balance the head directly over the spine, and directly over the feet. Our delicate necks are not made to hold that bowling-ball-head out in front of us, which is what happens when you sit with your feet out in front. If you are sitting at a computer with your feet in front of you, the tendency will be

4

to lean forward. Again, this is because the head is designed to rest directly over the feet as well as the hips and spine. With that heavy head leaning forward, the only thing keeping it from falling into your lap is – guess what – those hard working muscles at the back of your neck. Also straining are the muscles and tendons between your shoulder blades and across the top of your shoulders. Those are the very spots that hurt so much at the end of the workday. No wonder they get sore and tired! You feel like your head is too heavy – because it is! Your body wants your head to be effortlessly aligned over your center of gravity most of the time. So use the "Zip it Up" trick. It may take a few weeks of reminding yourself to make this correction a habit. Practice it in the car, when you're on the phone, whenever and wherever you think of it.

Back to chairs

My favorite seating option is a **'balance chair'**, or sometimes called a 'kneeling chair', and some companies call them an ergonomics chair. There are many variations of this chair; you may remember when they came out in the sixties, a Swedish invention, with a tilted seat and a knee rest. I find some of them do not function as well as others, and I have my favorite which is shown in the photo.

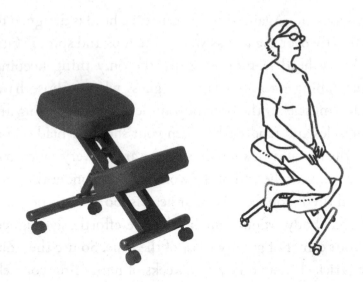

There is a description to help you find this chair online at the end of the book.

Most people look at these contraptions and hesitate to try them because it looks unsafe, as though you might fall out of it. (I've actually had people refuse them because their office mates will think they are weird!) It does not appear to have back support, so how could it be helpful?

Despite the misgivings, the chair actually does place your feet under you, which invites your head and body to balance comfortably over your center of gravity, as you do when you are standing. People think it will be work to balance this way, but once you try it you will find that it is actually an effortless position. Your knees rest lightly on the lower surface, and *Wa-lah!* You can sit this way *and* relax! It puts you naturally in the 'Zipped Up' alignment. I would say easily 98% of my clients with neck pain first sit in this chair and look at me in disbelief – because it feels so good. Their pain is immediately reduced. You will need to check to see if your desk is high enough for this chair to work for you. Or if needed you could put your keyboard and monitor on a higher surface. These chairs have a slight adjustability. It works fine with my short stature, and my tall male clients are very happy with it as well. Many of my clients have purchased this chair with excellent results. They are reasonably priced and of very good quality. I'd like to add that a couple of my clients with low back problems have used this chair both pre and post back surgery because it was the only way they could get comfortable.

If not a Balance Chair . . .

The other kind of seating that places you in a good position is a **barstool**. Taverns have had this figured out for centuries! If you sit in the middle of a bar stool and rest your feet on the rungs, you will notice that your feet are more under you. Your chest lifts, your torso lengthens, and your head balances easily on your neck. If you have a bar-height table in front of you, you may rest your arms on it. This posture should feel very comfortable. You may need to sit facing the corner of the stool if the seat is square, but find wherever it is that you are balanced, and your feet are under you. I've heard many clients exclaim to me, "Oh, so that's why I like to sit at the breakfast bar at home to work on my laptop!" Plus you can rest your forearms on the table to take pressure off of your shoulders. Another option is a **simple stool** you can get at the hardware store, or the type of stool you see your doctor sit on; which is round and has a platform to put feet on if you choose. Align yourself in the same way: Put your feet on the rungs under you and find yourself balanced. In my opinion, stools are very under-rated. Of course you'll want to have a cushion on it. Stools are great!

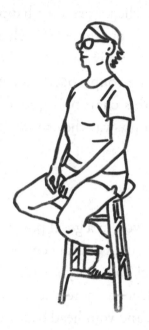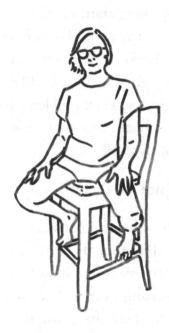

When in a kitchen chair you may find it comfortable to sit on the corner, knees apart and with your feet beneath you. If I am in a restaurant chair, I will have the chair pushed back and sit on the edge. Crazy? I don't think so! My torso is lengthened so food will digest more easily, my lungs will breathe more freely, and my neck will not hurt. I am upright and energized.

While I certainly have my chair preferences, I again want to emphasize that no chair is the right chair all of the time!

We need change, so I suggest using a balance chair or stool for a while, and then switch to a different chair. Use one for as long as you are comfortable, and then switch to a regular chair for a while-- all the while finding various ways to sit in each of them. Maybe you have office mates who would be willing to swap chairs now and then.

One of the best things you can do with a typical office chair is to sit forward toward the edge with your feet under you (or on the base if there is one.) When on the edge of a chair, kneeling chair or stool, one adjustment you can make periodically is to straighten one leg out to the side (or at the 2 o'clock direction), and the other foot under your center for a while. When you engage in this position, make sure that the heel of your straightened leg is on the floor. When it is again time to shift position, do the same with your other leg. By straightening one leg out to the side, the hamstrings will stretch. When your hamstrings shorten from sitting, it can be problematic for the lower back.

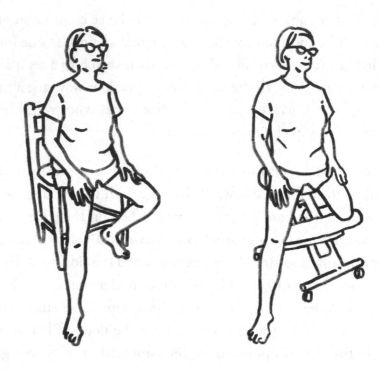

I am not in favor of arm rests on office chairs. If I put my arms on the arm rests, my shoulders likely hike up and in so doing the muscles across the top of my shoulders will shorten and stiffen. Plus they limit the possibility for me to move and stretch my arms around.

When in a traditional chair, you can put one foot out in front of you like usual, but always keep **at least one foot under you.** You could even cross your legs for a few minutes, as long as one foot is under you. I believe this only becomes problematic when it is done a lot of the time, and with the same leg. But for short periods, as long as one foot is under you, I think crossing legs is okay since it provides you with another option for change. (Some people have doctor's orders not to cross legs for various reasons, please follow your doctor's orders.) In general remember to alternate your leg positions often!

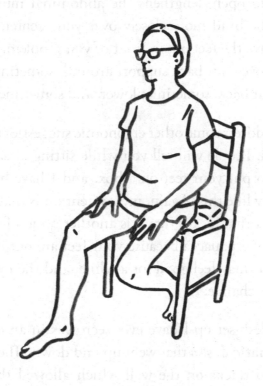

You may want to sit back in a regular chair for a while. I am not totally ruling out that that option. But again, it is just another option for a short time, and then you will need to change positions. If you must sit back in a chair, a couch, a car or plane seat, please have the back of the seat as close to upright as you can. You have got to get that head over your center! You want to prevent your head from jutting forward. Then there is something you can do to lengthen your torso. In these situations, putting a pillow or folded sweater behind your whole spine (not just your low back) can be helpful. I recommend placing a standard bed pillow behind people's spines. This provides a subtle shift in posture that causes the chest to open, lengthens the abdominal muscles, and balances the head more closely over your center, however, you still have the feet out in front of you problem. Also, it is good to move your back support around, sometimes higher behind your back, sometimes lower, and sometimes sit on it!

I want to address some other ergonomic suggestions you may have heard. People will tell you while sitting at a desk that it is best to put your feet on a box, and I have had clients tell me they like this. Again, my contention is that the good thing about that idea is that it is another option for change. But it is not a panacea because your feet are out in front of the spine. It may feel good for a while, and then your body will want a change.

The best desk set up I have ever seen was in an office that had **automatic desks** that went up and down. The desk was attached to tracks on the wall which allowed the user to stand while working, and as desired it could be put down to chair or stool level. I thought that solution was fabulous and hope it will be the wave of the future! I've recently seen free standing adjustable height desks now on the market, and I think it would be well worth the investment. The idea of the desk on a treadmill is novel, and I suppose periodically useful in the right circumstances. Fixed standing desks are available, but being limited to standing all day in place is not good for the low back.

Backwards: Another possibility, however unconventional and only appropriate in certain situations, is to sit backwards in a straight back chair. You may be able to pull this off in meetings, classes, and informal gatherings if you are wearing pants. Simply turn the chair around, straddle it and sit in it facing the back of the chair. Your knees will be bent so that your feet are partially planted on the floor at your sides lined up with your shoulders and hips. Try it, you'll see what I mean. This position encourages the torso to lengthen and the head to balance over spine. And then if you choose to rest your arms or hands on the chair back, it gives you a nice sense of taking the weight off of your shoulders. For another similar option, you may want to straddle this kind of chair even when sitting in a forward position.

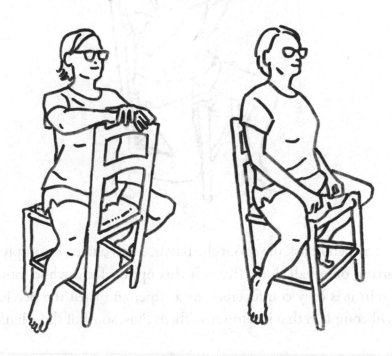

Recently I presented to a group of quilters. We discovered a good option for folks who do manual work at a table such as crafting, and even using a sewing machine. Sit facing forward with one foot out front and one leg off the side of the chair. The free leg bends back alongside of the chair, with that knee dropping toward the floor, and the ball of that foot rested on the floor in line with the hip. One could do this while on the computer as well.

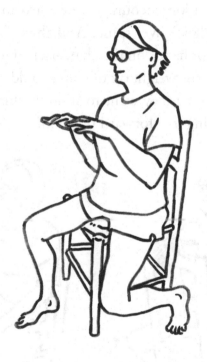

Many people ask me about the balance ball chairs, or simply sitting on a ball. I'm OK with this option for a while, but again it is only comfortable for a time, and then the pelvis will complain that it is too stretched. Plus, some of these ball chairs don't allow the feet to rest far enough back at your sides to be aligned with your hips and shoulders.

Living room seating: I am often asked if a recliner is ok. I think they are fine for a while, but you should add a pillow behind the back in order to lengthen the front of your torso, remember you want to avoid collapsing your front in any way for too long. If your legs are stretched out and your head is supported so that you are not straining to see the TV its ok, and you may need a small towel roll behind your neck for sufficient support and comfort. The same applies in a hospital bed. Whenever I visit someone in a hospital, where the bed head is tilted upward, I put a firm pillow behind them to lengthen the abdominal area.

Couches and lounge chairs are not usually great. These put your legs out in front and invite collapse of your front line. If you must sit in these situations, please put a substantial pillow behind the length of your spine so as to open the front of your torso. Try it, I think you'll like it! I do it wherever I go.

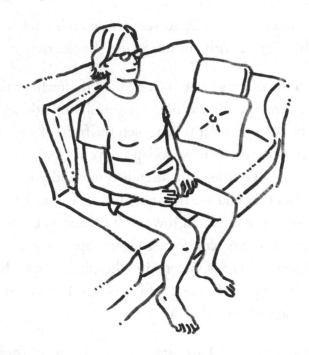

Sitting on the edge of a couch or bench where you can't get a foot under you can be done. Just turn sideways with your feet as close under your bottom as possible, and find your chest lifted. This is particularly good for a lady wearing a skirt. You may want to cross your ankles.

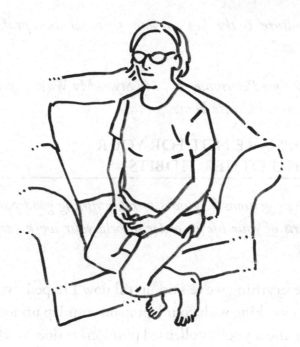

For a wonderful little video on seating and another alternative please go to You Tube and type in 'The Squat Song'.

"Your posture is the key to your personal and professional foundation."

—*Cindy Ann Peterson et al., My Style, My Way: Top Experts Reveal How to Create Yours.*

LAPTOPS ARE NOT FOR YOUR LAP, AND OTHER TIDBITS

Let these suggestions be guides to maintaining good posture in other parts of your life in order to help your work periods be easier.

*Given everything we've said up till now I hope it would be clear that working with your laptop on your lap undoubtedly puts you into a poorly collapsed position, as does working in bed. Best to put laptop on a table or on a high surface, like a pub table where you can stand or sit on a stool. If you want to work sitting on a couch or living room chair, you could put the laptop on a pillow in your lap. In that situation sit your butt way back, with a substantial pillow behind your back in order to perch your head over your center. Plus, change the position of your legs now and then from out front on an ottoman, to folded cross legged or otherwise. I don't recommend this for long periods of time.

*Don't bend over stuff if you can help it. When writing a check, place it on a high surface like at the bank counter or hold it up in front of your chest. When fishing around in your purse for something, hold it to your chest or waist instead of bending over it on a table. Try doing this by looking down with your **eyes**. Stand up while brushing your teeth and only bend forward when you have to rinse. When working on anything in front of you, stand close to it. For example when chopping veggies, stand close to or touching your belly to the counter. When picking something up from a table, take the extra step to get right next to the table instead of leaning over to reach it. I got a refrigerator that has the freezer on the bottom so that I don't bend over to get out the juice. I have a client who told me she puts her tablet in the cupboard so she doesn't lean over to use it.

*Speaking of purses, carry it **under your arm pit** in a relaxed way when you can. Or use one with a long enough strap to go around one side of your neck so that it crosses your body. Hanging it on one shoulder makes your shoulder muscles hike up and tighten. Obviously lightening the contents is always best.

*When you have to bend over to do something, always try to put one foot slightly forward, **soften your knees**, and keep your neck straight with your spine. That is what I do if I need to bend over my massage table to work, plus I extend one leg out behind as a counterweight. When I have to bend over to yank the door open to my dryer with my right hand, I brace my left hand on the dryer and kick my left leg out behind. As I pull on the door I slightly shift back to use my whole body to produce the force needed. It's like a dance, and the neck is still in a fairly straight line with my back.

*Supporting your head with your hands can be a good thing. For instance when you are sitting at a table listening to someone, or just reading the laptop, with your elbows on the table, rest your chin on your hands. This will work best if you are sitting on the edge of your chair and your torso is Zipped Up. When getting up from bed make it easier on your neck by supporting your head with your hand.

*Don't bend over to do something with two knees on the ground if you can help it. Rather, kneel on one knee and have the other foot on the ground out in front, and keep your neck straight with your back.

*Little children – I learned when I was teaching pre-school, that when I needed to help a child zip their jacket or talk to them face to face, it was far better to kneel. Have one foot forward on the floor, and the other knee on the floor. That way my back and neck were straight and I could maintain my 'Zip Up position". And if you are tying their shoe, the knee in front of you can serve as a "lean-to"; this is also very good for weeding in the garden.

*Put your work in front of you. For assembling projects, sharpening the lawn mower, potting plants, put it on a table instead of bending to the ground. Put the grocery bag on the counter next to the fridge, instead of on the floor to unpack. There will be enough times when we must compromise our posture, so don't do it if you can find another way.

*To tie your shoe, slip it onto your foot on the floor and then perch it up on a higher surface to tie it, like on the edge of a counter, or as I do on the corner of my low dresser. No bending your head over to do it on the floor or with it crossed over your knee.

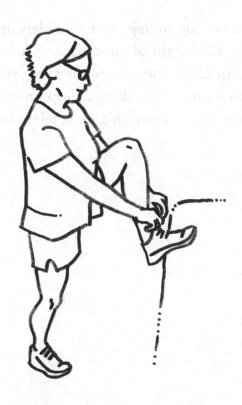

*Watch your nodding. I see lots of folks who nod their heads a lot. Each time the head goes forward, the neck muscles have to tighten to stop it and bring it back. Doing this repeatedly causes undo stress on your neck. When we nod it is usually because we are acknowledging that we agree with or hear the person we are talking to. We can instead relax and know that our eye contact tells them we are listening. Besides, if you are in the Zipped Up position, you will find that rigorous nodding isn't possible, and instead it becomes a gentle, small movement.

*Be aware if you are hiking your shoulders up, and think about feeling the weight of your arms to help them come down. For a quick fix you can simply shrug your shoulders way up to your ears while taking a deep breath, and as you exhale feel them drop down in a more relaxed way.

"Our bodies change our minds, and our minds can change our behavior, and our behavior can change our outcomes, we can even change our own body chemistry."

Amy Cuddy – American social psychologist and Body Language Researcher

PECTORAL STRETCHING

The pectoral muscle is the muscle that moves your arm in front of you. It goes from sternum in the middle of your chest and from under the collar bone, to the front of your upper arm. It is the major muscle that pulls your arm forward for doing any task, which we do so much of the time every day, all of our lives!

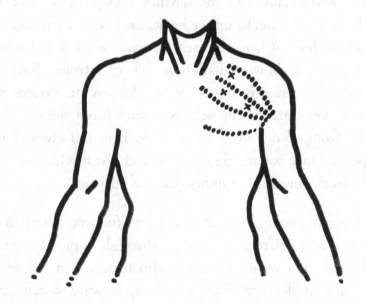

In order to counteract the collapse in the front of our body, we need to open up across the chest whenever possible. Daily tasks that require using arms in front of us all shorten the 'pects'. This includes picking things up, chopping food, hammering nails, folding and lifting laundry, carrying groceries and children, driving, playing instruments, working on cars, cutting hair, washing everything, and of course holding arms in position to type and mouse for hours. The more we do these things, those pectorals become stuck in a shortened position. And in time we begin to see permanently inward rounded shoulders, and likely the head jutting out frontward. Nature takes up the slack in shortened muscles which is why these repeated actions leave us with short pectorals.

The point of addressing this area oddly enough, is because it is **directly related to the tension and pain we feel in the back of the neck, upper back, and across the top of the shoulders**. When we reach forward, what muscles are holding up our 'bowling ball' head to keep it from falling in our lap? The answer is those very muscles just mentioned; no wonder they hurt! So the need is to stretch out the muscles in the front of our body in order to help ourselves align properly. Once we are aligned, the end result will ease the stress on the posterior muscles that are hurting.

My favorite pectoral stretch is done as follows: Stand in a doorway as if you're going to walk through it, put the hand of the side you want to stretch palm forward on the door frame at shoulder level. Next, take a step forward so that that arm is straight and behind you with your hand hooked on the door frame. Now lean forward **gently.** Feel the stretch up your inner arm and across your pectoral (chest) muscles. If it is painful to do this with your hand at shoulder height, you can do it with your hand lower on the frame to begin with. Then eventually over time move your hand up a little higher each day. You may feel the stretch down into your forearm which is fine because stretching those muscles will also help prevent carpal tunnel syndrome. It takes around thirty seconds for a muscle to stretch, so stay there for thirty seconds to a minute or longer if you like. Be extra cautious here, you could eventually throw your shoulder out by pulling too hard, so be careful not to do anything that hurts. This should be a gentle, easy task and feel good. After the stretch the important thing is to <u>take a minute</u> to stand with your arm hanging down and <u>feel</u> the effect of the stretched arm and pectoral. You may notice that your neck feels more comfortable now, and that you are standing straighter. **Take time** for your body and mind to register the change before you go back to your work.

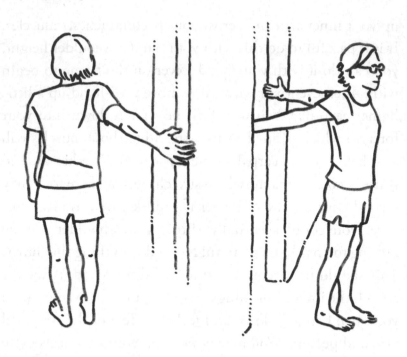

You can address both arms at the same time by doing the same thing but with one hand on each side of the door frame, however I find it more effective to do one side at a time. Try to do this for at least thirty seconds periodically through the day especially if you are at the computer for long hours. If there is not time to go stand in the doorway, you can reach back with both arms, clasp hands behind you and if possible lift them toward the ceiling. This can be done sitting or standing. This is SO important, and it should feel oh so good!

If you have one of those big balls that are from knee height to hip height, lay back on it. Let your head lay back and extend arms out to the sides, and rest there. Two minutes in this position will leave you standing straight and feeling like a new person! Feel the gentle stretch across your chest, and down the front of your arms and wrists, even into fingers.

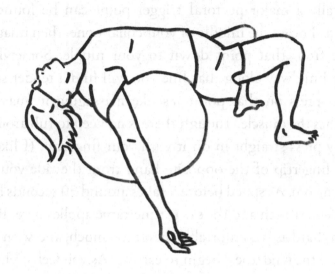

Rice bags: My clients love this – Lay on your back and put a 10 pound bag of rice on each shoulder/pectoral area. Rest with this for at least a few minutes. This will help to passively stretch those pectoral muscles as well as sending a message to your neck that it's time to rest and let go.

PECTORAL TRIGGER POINTS:

And lastly, you can work the trigger points in your pectoral muscles to release tension there and help your neck. Trigger points are little areas in muscles where overuse has caused acidic buildup, agitated nerves and hypertonicity. When you press on one of these spots forcefully it will hurt. You can find many trigger points in your pectoral muscle by walking your fingers around on the muscle, and notice where it feels tender.

Typically a major pectoral trigger point can be found as follows: Locate the middle of your collar bone, then imagine a line from that point down to your nipple. Somewhere around midway along that line you will find a tender spot. If you press on that point it's like massaging it, massage stretches the muscle. Though there is no need to rub around, simply press straight in on it with your fingertip. (I like to use a fingertip of the opposite hand from the side you are working on). As stated before it takes around 30 seconds for a muscle to stretch and the same timeframe applies here. Press only as hard as is comfortable, never too much, and soon you will feel the tenderness begin to ease up. As you feel it release, you can then press a little harder for another 30 seconds, or else walk your fingers around and find another spot to treat. Notice after you have done this if the pain in your neck or upper back has subsided. You can do this at any time in your day while at the computer, driving or sitting in a meeting. I like to do it as I lie in bed on my side.

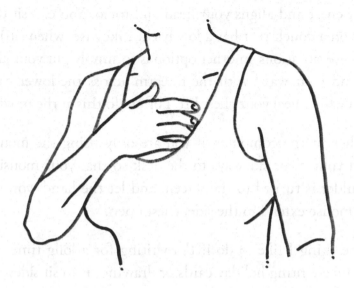

On the same note, think about other ways to **open your chest in daily life**.

* For example, if it is safe when you are **driving,** sometimes put your right arm behind or on top of the back of the passenger seat for a few minutes. Alternately, since you can't do that with your left arm, what you **can** do is to reach your left hand up and back and hold on to the head rest. These actions will put your head directly over your spine, and lengthen your torso up out of "the forward collapse". Your neck will love this; I figured it out driving across country and it really made all the difference! (Of course you can only do one arm at a time as you are steering, please!)

*If you are in a theater or church, put your arm(s) across the back of the seat or bench next to you. You see people doing this all the time, and it's exactly because it feels good, opens your chest and aligns your head and torso. You can sit this way on a couch that has a low back. Likewise, when sitting in these situations, another option is to simply put your arm behind your waist with the forearm across the lower back for a while. Feel your chest lift. I often do this at the movies.

*When at the computer, if you are only using the mouse, turn your chair sideways to the desk so that your mousing shoulder is turned to the screen, and let the hand working the mouse extend to the side, chest open.

*One thing I like to do if I'm writing for a long time, for instance writing holiday cards or drawing, is to sit sideways to the desk or table. If you are right handed, turn the chair so it is next to the desk facing left, with your writing hand/ shoulder next to the desk. This posture allows your writing hand to be out to the side, arm resting on the table. The right side of your chest and shoulder are opened up, which is so important. So rather than bending forward your head is upright and only slightly bent to the right, and your eyes looking are down to the paper. And while you are taking good care of yourself with these new positions, please also remember to relax your jaw!

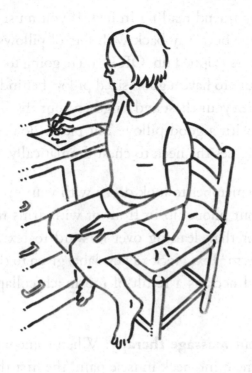

Reading:

Generally, the goal is to keep from collapsing forward. In any situation, try to hold the reading material up high enough in front of you so that your head doesn't have to bend down.

At home, try sitting sideways on the couch, legs curled, and prop the book or tablet on the back of the couch **at eye level** to keep from looking down. In this position take a moment to appreciate the nice stretch of your side against the couch, and the long 'Zipped Up' organization of your torso. You may want a pillow between your side and the couch. Switch sides now and then and periodically stretch legs out.

I don't recommend reading in bed. If you must do this, sit up with your butt way back with lots of pillows behind to keep your torso zipped up. OR if you're going to do it laying down, be sure to have a good sized pillow behind your spine that will open your chest and lengthen your abs. Then bolster your neck with a good pillow. But please don't do this for long, it collapses the neck to chest dramatically.

Texting: Remember to look down with your eyes, or better yet hold your phone up in front or with arms resting on a table, rather than leaning over forward to text. I recently heard the term 'Text Neck', a new label given to the situation of a painful neck as a result of too much collapsing while texting.

A note about **massage therapy**: When someone comes to me with screaming neck muscle pain, the first thing I do is to work on the shortened pectoral and abdominal muscles. Most folks think when their neck is hurting I should work on muscles at the back of their neck, which sounds logical. But think about it, if I work the muscles on the back of the neck, it is going to lengthen those muscles. Longer posterior neck muscles will result in the head falling forward in greater collapse. It may feel good at the time, but in the end prolongs the problem. What is usually needed is to release the short, tight, hardworking muscles on the front of the body. Thus, you can more easily stand upright and balanced where the neck is happy. I've seen this work over and over. Then I may work a little on the posterior, or back of the neck muscles just because it feels good, but my primary goal is to release those abdominal and pectoral muscles that pull the neck and upper body forward.

Eye Exercise - Lately I'm hearing new information about how our constant staring at computers and TV eventually weakens eye muscles. When we look straight ahead so much of the time, the outer eye muscles lose their ability to contract fully and smoothly in different directions. The effects of this occurrence are numerous. One outcome is that it begins to limit our full body movement in general because we typically look with our eyes in the direction we are moving. Our eyes inform our brains and bodies to perform a multitude of tasks. You can find instructions for doing eye exercises online. The simplest way is to periodically practice shifting your eyes up, down, side to side and circling around the perimeter of your eye sockets, all without moving your head.

"I want to grow old gracefully. I want to have good posture, I want to be healthy and be an example to my children." Sting

LENGTHEN TORSO

A few of the chest opening suggestions also include lengthening of the abdominal area. It is important to see how this is also connected to neck and back discomfort. Notice that when you sit, the tendency is for the space at your waist to shorten or collapse. Remember, when muscles shorten nature takes up the slack. Believe it or not your belly muscles will begin to retain that shortness after hours of sitting. You may want to pay attention here because the shortening of your torso in this way leads to the pooching out of your not so welcomed 'love handles'. Again the remedy here is to 'Zip Up' effortlessly, which happens to lengthen abdominal muscles and align your spine.

Other ways to **Lengthen the Torso:**

*We've all seen someone sitting in an office chair leaning back with their hands interlaced behind their head and elbows out to the sides, I love it! I've heard it referred to as a 'power position', and it's a great abdominal stretch.

*Lie back on a large plastic ball, or ottoman, as was suggested for chest opening.

*Lie across the bed with your head almost hanging over the edge, arms out to the sides, and feel the stretch of your abdomen.

*Avoid crossing arms in front of you. Many people are in the habit of this stance, but it clearly invites collapse of the chest, shoulders, and abdomen, and likely brings the head forward. Instead it's much better to clasp hands behind your lower body, still with chest Zipped Up. Another good alternative is standing with hands on hips, facing either up or down are both fine.

Alternative to Sit Ups

Sit ups are awful, we don't like doing them and I'll tell you why. (For our purposes I include any kind of crunches and even leg lifts in this discussion). The problem with sit ups is that they shorten the long abdominal muscles that go from your ribs to pelvis in front. This is exactly what brings your body into forward collapse. If you shorten these muscles doing sit ups, they will be continually pulling your chest and head down. Then your posterior neck and back muscles will have to constantly fight to counteract that pull, making them tired and tight.

Instead we need to strengthen the transverse abdominal muscles which act like a girdle drawing your mid-section <u>in</u>. **Stretch your arms over head while standing or lying, and suck your belly in tight.** It's as simple as that. You can do this for repeated short bursts, or hold for several seconds. Do it however long and however strongly you like to do it. This action pulls your ribs up away from the pelvis, which is what you want. It gives more vertical space for digestive organs, strengthens transverse and other core muscles, and provides support to lower back, and is safe for the neck. (Some people will say they need to do their sit ups for their back. A teacher of mine said the only reason sit ups can help a back feel good is because it is movement and the back needs to have movement. We hear that people find they need to do the sit ups every day to help their back; in the long run it doesn't cure the problem). I'm ok with yoga Plank position for core strengthening, though again the neck must be straight with spine and for a short time.

"Good posture is not a position, it's a direction. Life energy floating the body up away from gravity." – Roger Tolle, Trager® Instructor

FOR YOUR LOW BACK AND QUADRICEPS STRETCHING

Typically the reason for minor low back pain begins with the shortening of anterior muscles, or muscles on the front of your body. Think of when you are bending over for any length of time, for example pulling weeds. At some point your low back begins to rebel. You try to stand up but your low back hurts and it's hard to straighten up. In the same way, when we sit at the computer for any length of time it can be hard to straighten up as we stand. What has happened is that in your bending over #1) the muscles of your low back have been over working. They tighten to keep your heavy upper body and head from falling forward as you bend over, and #2) the muscles on the front of your body – the abs, the psoas (deep on the front of your spine), and your quadriceps (the front thigh muscles), all **shorten during your bending and sitting**. So as nature takes up the slack, those shortened anterior muscles are fixed in the tight position. Thus when you try to straighten up, the tense front muscles are basically fighting the effort of your back muscles to pull you upright. That in turn makes your back work harder and it hurts even more. As discussed earlier, the same thing happens when you've been sitting in traditional seating at the desk, school, or in the car. It hurts to get up.

What can you do to alleviate low back pain in these instances? Again, the answer is to lengthen the front, 'Zip Up'. Always remember, you can stretch your abdominal muscles simply by reaching your arms over head and stretching up, without arching your low back. Lift to make space between the ribs and pelvis. And very importantly:

Stretch Quadriceps – It is most important for low back health that you stretch the muscles on the front of your thigh! These hard working muscles shorten when we sit, bend, run and lift. They are attached to the front of your pelvis and when tight they pull your pelvis down in front which in turn pulls on and shortens the lower back which can be painful.

One way to do this stretch is to grab a foot behind you with your hand while standing or laying on your side, and gently pull that foot toward your bottom. Try to keep your knees as close together as is comfortable. Please note that if this is not possible, or is uncomfortable at first for your knee or your low back, then start out smaller. For example rest your foot behind you on the bottom rung of a stool, or on the seat of a chair as you hold a wall or something for stability. Be careful not to arch your back. Some of my clients like to grasp the back of their pant leg instead of their foot, and then pull up in the same way. Give this stretch thirty seconds or so and then do it with the other leg. You should feel a gentle stretch on the front of your thigh, nothing should hurt. Then again after the stretch, stand still for a minute and feel the change. Notice if your back feels better and let your body/mind remember this.

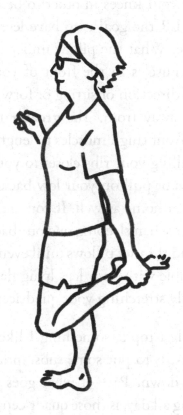

Of course the other way to stretch the anterior muscles of the abdomen or thigh is to massage them, or work the trigger points which may require finding a good massage therapist.

Note – Often when we go see a massage therapist, chiropractor or other health professional for low back pain, one of the first things they do is put a pillow or bolster under your knees when you lie on your back. At first glance this seems to make sense since it helps your low back to rest down on the table and it feels good. I take issue with this habit. What I tell my clients is, "By all means if you need to have a support under your knees in order to be comfortable let's do it, HOWEVER the goal is to have legs straight here as much as possible. What the pillow under the knees does is shortening the muscles in the front of your body. It puts you in the same direction of sitting or forward collapse that we want to get away from. The **greater** need is for your abdominal and front thigh muscles to lengthen, in order for them to stop pulling your ribs closer to your legs. This will lead to less stress or pull on your low back. I ask clients to be aware of this at home as well. If you are used to a pillow under your knees when sleeping on your back, try gradually using thinner and thinner pillows until eventually your back can be comfortable with your legs lying flat. (Along with a program of gently stretching your quadriceps.)

Related to that last topic, something I like to do with low back pain clients, is to put some substantial weight on the lap while lying down. Part of what goes on when we lie down after sitting all day, is those quadriceps muscles are still shortened. If we put a pillow across the lap in lying position, and place a couple of heavy weights, say ten or fifteen pounds per leg, on top of the pillow it encourages the quadriceps to lengthen out. And what's more is it sends a strong message to the low back that says, "Hey, were stuck here now, were done with our day, I can't get up, so might as well just relax!" I hope you will try this. Our poor backs are so used to being at the ready to jump up and answer the call, we go to bed being all wound up and those hard working muscles forget how to relax.

Other low back hints . . .

*Soften your **knees, never lock them** when standing. I would say almost 90% of the clients I see who lock their knees have low back pain. It's not that you have to bend your knees, just soften them, and don't push them back into a stiff position.

*Stand and walk with feet parallel and near hip width apart.

*When standing, shift your weight from side to side, never standing stiff while waiting in a line.

*When sitting on the edge of the chair, occasionally straighten each leg out to the side alternately for a while to stretch hamstrings. Change chairs now and then.

*Do a gentle kick walk. Just a meandering walk, giving a gentle kick with every step forward. See if you can feel a vibration reverberate up your thigh, gluteal muscles, pelvis, low back and spine. Enjoy the movement.

*Press trigger points in your lateral quadriceps muscles, (outside-front of thigh). Just like with the pectoral trigger points, find a tender spot, press for thirty seconds or more, not too hard, not too soft. Notice if any discomfort in your low back releases.

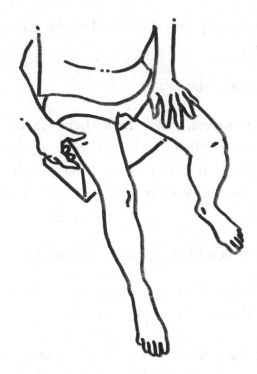

I have a client who actually rolls a rolling pin along the front and outer top edge of her thigh to get the muscles to soften. This gives her great relief during intense hours at the computer.

*And at the end of the day sit on the edge of the bed and lay back to stretch quads and abs. (You may want a small pillow under your low back with this).

*Use a pillow between knees when sleeping on your side. This is particularly good for the pelvis and hips.

For your Knees

*Stretch the hamstrings on the back of your thigh by leaning over with your hands or arms on a counter, and go slightly sway back. You can then shift your hips backward gently to get a deeper hamstring stretch. Careful not to overstretch.

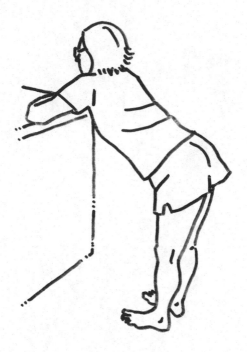

And as mentioned earlier, when sitting, stretch your legs out to the side regularly. One might think that sitting would stretch hamstrings, but in fact it actually shortens them. This is because the hamstrings wrap around from the back of the thigh and attach below the knee in front. So the effect of bending the knees, as in sitting, shortens the hamstrings. Of course we get the same shortening when sitting in a kneeling chair, and that is why I've suggested straightening the legs alternately off to the side now and then while in any chair.

"Happiness is not a matter of intensity but of balance and order and rhythm and harmony."

Thomas Merton, No Man Is An Island.

SLEEPING AND PILLOWS

One of my teachers said, "If you are truly relaxed, you can sleep in any position you like and you will be fine." But the problem is that more commonly we take our tension to bed with us and don't even realize it. Have you ever wakened in the middle of the night with neck or hip pain, and had difficulty falling back to sleep because of it? The bottom line is that pain is very often a result of your tension habits. It's hard to let go of our tension in this day and age, but one of the most beneficial things you can do for body and mind is to do some sort of relaxation practice before bedtime. Whether you do some gentle yoga, deep breathing, stretching, meditation, or a guided imagery where you visualize your muscles relaxing and feel the weight of each body part, these can all make for a more restful sleep. I don't recommend reading in bed because generally there is not a good position for your neck to do this without collapsing forward. Besides, as experts have been telling us for some time, to make for good restful sleep remember, the bed is for two things: sleeping and love making; not for watching TV, doing homework, texting or worrying.

Again, as in everything, I also apply the rule of change to sleeping. It's fine to move around in your sleep so not to get stuck in a position. I do have some postural suggestions you might like to try for sleeping.

<u>Back Sleeping</u>: Generally laying on your back is great if you have a fairly firm mattress that doesn't cave in, and you don't use thick pillows under your head. Ideally to keep your torso open when on your back, it's best to use a thin pillow if any. Try adding a bit of support under your neck like the edge of the pillow rolled up or a towel roll that fits the hollow of your neck. This lets the head fall back rather than pushed forward into a collapsed position by too thick a pillow. I'm not real keen on the idea of a pillow under your knees in this position. If you absolutely need to have a pillow under your knees for your low back to be comfortable then do it. Though remember, the goal is to help the front of your torso be long and open, so bending your hips in any degree is not best. You may like to rest your arms overhead which is fine for a while because it lengthens your abs, though too much of this will shorten the muscles across the tops of your shoulders and could cause trouble.

<u>Side Sleeping:</u> Pillows, pillows, pillows! Stay away from the fetal position where your head is bent forward, hips and knees folded in and shoulders and arms collapsed inward. Your neck wants your head to be positioned back a little on the pillow so it is straight with your spine. Shoulders should be open with the top arm resting on your side or hip. If you find that difficult, rest that arm on a large pillow in front of your torso. Here again it's best to have legs as straight as possible, with a pillow between thighs and knees which

keeps the hips from collapsing. You may be thinking this is a lot of pillows, but if it means staying out of pain it's worth it! Lastly, remember to feel the weight of your head on the pillow. If I take my tension with me to bed, it happens that even though my head is on the pillow, I will still be holding my head in position out of habit. I need first to be aware that I'm doing that, and then to consciously feel the weight (of my bowling ball head), and let it give in to gravity on the pillow. You could even rest your arm on your head to signal it to let go. Imagine a sleeping baby, or puppy and allow yourself to drift.

Side Pillow: If you suffer with neck pain please try this: Situate yourself on your side and add a **thin** pillow under the side you are lying on, from waistline to armpit or whatever you find to be comfortable. (I use a squishy down pillow here). To explain why this is good I want you to imagine how your heavy spine sinks down when you are on your side, and see how having a thin pillow there helps to raise that spine up, making a more horizontal line from neck to pelvis. I can't emphasize enough the importance of having your neck straight with your spine. Note: If you use this arrangement, make sure you have a good thick pillow, or two thin ones under your head so that neck is not bent down. This position also keeps your low back straight where it attaches to the pelvis. Many people have told me this position has alleviated their neck pain and some have resolved headache pain.

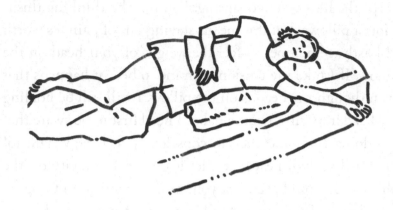

<u>Stomach Sleeping:</u> Not a good idea. This position cranks your neck in some bad way, and probably compromises your jaw. If you are hopelessly addicted to this position as I often am, at least have a thick pillow under the shoulder your head is facing to take stress off of your neck and jaw. Adding the thin pillow under your torso will also support your low back here.

<u>Switch Pillows:</u> We need to change pillows now and then. I have two favorite head pillows that I go back and forth with. And I don't just make the switch regularly, but rather I let my body tell me when it needs a different set up. When one pillow stops working well, I try another. Sometimes I find that although I feel comfortable I'm not sleeping well, which alerts me to make a change, I switch pillows and often sleep returns.

<u>Types of Pillows:</u> People ask me about cervical pillows, or the special pillow they bought after seeing it on TV. I like the cervical pillow; you'll need to spend a bit extra to get a good

quality one. These are the pillows with thicker edges and a dip in the middle. One edge is thicker for supporting your neck while lying on the side, and the other edge is less thick for under your neck while lying on the back. Sometimes I use the cervical pillow when side sleeping, but I add a thin pillow under it so that it's high enough for me. I think any of these pillows are fine, it's about personal preference. Just remember that it's helpful to change pillows when you are ready.

Other Alternatives:

Lying on a Long Pillow: **A Very Important Therapeutic Option**

This is a position I generally give people to help relieve tension when they get home from work or school for a few minutes. There would be nothing wrong with sleeping this way for a while if you like, or just do it for the first ten minutes you lay down at night. I've seen numerous clients come in close to tears with upper back or neck pain, who find great relief in this position, and after they do it. (Note: If you have bulging discs or nerve impingement, this may or may not be helpful.)

*Lay back lengthwise on a king sized pillow, or you can use two standard pillows placed end to end. Lay so that your neck is fully supported on the end of the pillow and your head is partly falling back over the end. Make sure your tail bone is fully on the pillow in order to avoid arching of the low back. What is good about this situation is that it causes a passive stretch of the pectoral or chest muscles because your arms hang off the sides, and it lengthens the abdominal muscles. Plus your heavy 'bowling ball' head is hanging slightly over the end to the degree that your neck is forced to let go of its tension because it can't even try to hold that head up. That sends a strong signal to your neck to let go and relax. (My clients with neck pain and headaches especially appreciate this position). It is important here to think of the weight of your head falling back, or sinking down. Play with the thickness of pillows you lie on and find what works for you. I love lying back on a thick king size pillow this way. You may also want to add a small towel roll under your neck as well.

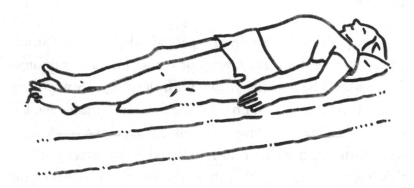

A simple variation of this position would be to lay across your bed with the top of your head slightly hanging over the edge, and arms stretched out to the sides. Add a small folded towel under your low back if you like.

<u>Laced Fingers on Forehead</u>

This is a little trick I've recently discovered for the neck. Do this while lying on your back either flat or on a long pillow as described in the last section. Lace the fingers of both hands and rest the back of them on your forehead across your eyebrows, or wherever it feels comfortable. Then just let the weight of your arms hang, elbows out to the sides. Spend a few minutes this way until you feel your neck relax. Feel the opening of your chest and your belly lengthening. What happens is the weight of your hands sends a message to your neck that says, "Wow this head is so heavy, I can't even think about holding it up; we're not going anywhere and all I can do is relax." The deep muscles of the neck will give up their habit of constant tension. This can also be helpful for tension headache pain.

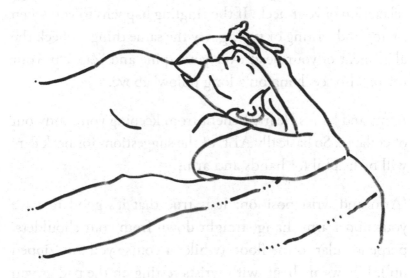

For Arms and Hands

Numbness, or Tingling Pain

Do you ever wake up with these symptoms? Most often I find this is due to neck position. In sleeping, if you are tense and your neck is bent forward or sideways, or any way that is not straight with your spine, it can cause muscles to impinge on the nerves that feed your arm or hand, which can cause the discomfort. When this happens I find that repositioning my head so that the neck is straight with my spine will usually relieve the pain within a few minutes. In bed feel the weight of your head sinking into the pillow in order to encourage relaxation of your neck. If the tingling happens to you when sitting and writing or typing, try the same thing – check the alignment of your head over your spine and 'Zip Up' your torso. Also see 'lying on a long pillow' above.

Arms and hands clearly benefit from keeping your body out of collapse. So basically ALL of the suggestions for neck care will be helpful for hands and arms.

*Arm and wrist position: It is true that it's good to have your upper arms hang straight down from your shoulders, perpendicular to the floor, (while of course you are 'zipped up'). Elbows are bent, with wrists resting on the pad as you type. However, again change is good, and that may mean moving the keyboard height down periodically. I have my laptop on a pub table with bar stool, so sometimes I move the whole thing farther away with my forearms resting on the table for a while which takes the weight off of my shoulders.

As other ergonomic manuals will tell you, it is best to have your wrists straight with your forearms while typing most of the time.

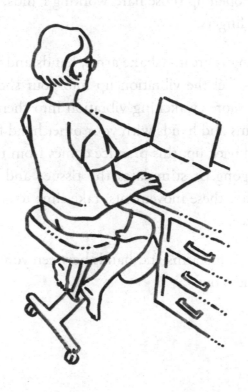

*Your hold on the mouse needs to be light. Some people have an unconscious habit of gripping the mouse tightly which tenses not only the hand and wrist but the whole arm and shoulder.

*When doing the pectoral stretch, be aware of the gentle stretch also reaching into the inner forearm and wrist. This can help prevent carpel tunnel problems.

*You can stretch the inside of your hands and fingers by gently pressing them palms open on the edge of counter tops, on the roof of the car, on the head of your bed, or on your thighs. Just open up those hard working hands, and wiggle and stretch fingers.

*Also shaking is great – shake arms, hands and fingers out, up, down – feel the vibration up into your shoulders and neck. Send more awakening vibration into them by gently slapping arms and hands with your other hand from top to bottom and back up; this practice comes from the Chinese art of chi gong. It stimulates the tissues and gets blood moving. After these movements, take time to stop and feel the difference.

*Squeeze your forearms and hands between your knees as if wringing them out.

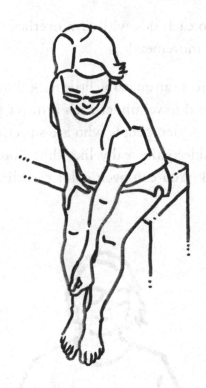

*These are all things you can do while sitting at the computer. And remember the rule of change, change the height of your keyboard and computer screen. If you have a portable coffee tray or tall stool, place it next to you and put the mouse on it so that for a while you can work the mouse from a position of an opened chest and shoulder.

*Think of your arms hanging softly from your shoulders like a porch swing hanging from the hinges.

*Stand up and with arms dangling loosely, twist your torso from side to side, letting your arms fling freely as if they were limp noodles.

*Stretch over to each side with arm overhead when you sit, do any kind of movement!

*Pit Pillows – Here's an amazing little trick. Put a small pillow or rolled up hand towel under each arm pit periodically as you are typing. Often people who are suffering with upper back and shoulder pain really like this. Sounds crazy, see what you think. You can even color coordinate with your wardrobe!

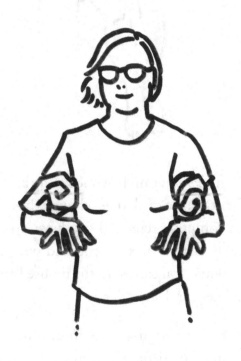

(Note – I am not fully knowledgeable about key boards and wrist supports so will not address those in this manual, but again I do suggest occasional change with those things as well).

*Lastly, remember to BREATHE!!! Breathe length into your torso, and breathe oxygen into your back and extremities. Then Feel your Weight in your Seat! Watch your sense of urgency, you can only do what you can do in the moment. I'm fond of telling clients to remember – in the car, you'll get there just as fast by relaxing, settling back and pressing the gas pedal, as you would if you're frantically leaning forward and gripping the wheel! BREATHE and feel the Present!!!!

"Life is like riding a bicycle. To keep your balance, you must keep moving."

Albert Einstein in a letter to his son Eduard, February 5, 1930.
©Albert Einstein Archives / The Hebrew University of Jerusalem

GENERAL SUPPORTING SELF CARE

We all know by now that there are many things we can and need to be doing to take care of our bodies and minds regardless of the demands of our work situation. I want to briefly mention a few here.

MOVE of course!!!

I'm always glad when clients assure me that they get up from their desk every half hour and stretch a little, or take the stairs several times a day, or walk to the copy machine periodically. May I add . . . try a little jog to the drinking fountain or the bathroom. I do that at home. When did we get so grown up as to forget that as children we ran down the hall when we could just because it felt good, and it's good for us? Why save it for an appointed hour a few times per week at the gym? We need to get the circulation and adrenalin moving as much as possible through the day to prevent early aging, muscle atrophy and other problems.

You can find all sorts of videos on exercises to do at the desk. While sitting, periodically get your arms up overhead, circle the wrists and shoulders, all while breathing deeply. Stretch your legs out, circle ankles, stretch your sides. Fitting exercise into our day is key to our wellbeing and some sort of cardio activity is most beneficial. I like the Aging Backwards Classical Stretch DVDs by Marinda Esmond White. Or look up You Tube videos of Trager Mentastics® for gentle self-help movement to free your muscles of unwanted tension. Do things that you enjoy; if you can't get to a gym then put on some music and dance, or play catch with a buddy, or my favorite – throw a Frisbee. Of course walking is fabulous, be sure to keep your 'Zip Up' going on!

Relaxation

Find ways to balance activity and rest in your day. Make time for meditation, or yoga, soothing relaxation music, Tai Chi or whatever works for you, even if for only fifteen minutes. Periodically through the day consciously send messages of relaxation to your body. Think of dropping your shoulders. Notice how the 'Zip Up' posture takes stress away, then soften your face, and drop your jaw. You can periodically take mini rest breaks throughout the day by closing your eyes, letting your arms hang, feeling your weight in the seat, taking a deep breath and for a moment appreciate the ease and calm you can give yourself. To set yourself up for a good night's sleep, give yourself twenty minutes of gentle stretching, relaxed movement or focused breathing before going to bed.

There are numerous mind/body modalities that promote relaxation, movement awareness and centeredness as well as good posture. I have been a Practitioner and tutor of **The Trager Approach®** for 30 years. Trager work is a profound yet soft approach to body/mind tension pattern release that is different from massage. It can be helpful for stress management, pain control, fibromyalgia, sleep and digestive disorders, anxiety, rheumatoid arthritis, headaches and more. To enhance well-being, increase range of motion and reduce muscle stiffness, Trager uses gentle rocking and swinging movement, stretching, pressing and soothing touch. Trager practitioners teach self-care movements that show the body and mind what it is to feel lighter, freer, and more open in your body.

A few other favorites of mine are The Feldenkrais Method®, Body-Mind Centering®, The Alexander Technique, and NIA; and there are many more. For more information see: www.trager.com, www.feldenkrais.com, www.bodymindcentering.com, www.alexandertechnique.com, and NIAnow.com.

Nutrition & Water

Giving your body the right kind of fuel is so important. As I'm sure you know eating fresh fruits and vegetables, proteins and whole grains, organic if possible, supports all systems including bones, nerves, digestion and brain as well as muscles. Staying away from too many carbs, sugary drinks and processed foods helps get us through the day with less of the afternoon slump where we give in to the postural collapse.

One can't say enough about drinking water. 75% of Americans are chronically dehydrated. Lack of water is a big trigger for afternoon fatigue. I've heard preliminary research indicates that 8-10 glasses of water a day could significantly ease back and joint pain for up to 80% of sufferers. A mere 2% drop in body water can trigger fuzzy short term memory, trouble with basic math, and difficulty focusing on the computer screen. Make it a habit to have your water bottle at your work station, and please drink it!

Get outside

Whenever you can, get yourself out in nature and drink it in! It is a nourishing tonic for our mind, body and soul, even if only to look up at the sky and feel the air on your skin.

Breathe

Breathing fully not only gets oxygen to your brain, blood, organs and tissues. It energizes, helps manage stress, relaxes, calms anxiety and supports alertness. Breathing is a key mechanism in successful digestion and elimination. If you are sitting at a desk most of the day then you must take deep breaths often and develop a habit of deep breathing while you work. Your abdomen should expand and contract with each breath, like a baby. For further instruction in proper breathing look it up online, there are many excellent videos on YouTube about belly breathing.

REMINDER LIST OF HELPFUL HINTS – FOR QUICK REFERENCE

Posture, Rule # 1 ZIP IT UP to stay out of collapse!

The goal is for your head to be balanced over the center of your skeleton. It's not about pulling your head back. Rather Zip Up your sternum, as in zipping up your jacket, with shoulders relaxed and chin level. Do this while standing, sitting, walking, driving and working as much as possible.

<u>Sitting</u> Yes – chairs and couches are bad!

*It's best to sit on a kneeling chair, a stool, or on the edge of a chair with one or both feet under you. Or you can sit on the side of a stool with one foot on the floor, changing sides now and then.

*Extend your legs out to the side one at a time periodically to gently stretch hamstrings.

*Think of your arms hanging softly from your shoulders. Think of them as a porch swing.

*Sometimes you can rest your arms and elbows extended out front on the table for a while with the keyboard or laptop farther away, **as long as you are Zipped Up!**

*If sitting in a couch or car, put a pillow behind your back. Periodically move it up or down, sometimes sit on it. You may like to use a folded towel in the car, so you can make it different sizes.

*When you can, sit backwards in a straight chair.

For Your Neck

*Zip It Up!

*Pectoral stretches in door frame. Gently stretching inner arms and hands too. Or simply clasp hands behind you and lift them upward.

*Press trigger points in chest muscles, (pectorals).

*In standing, clasp hands behind you, rather than crossing arms in front.

*When leaning over, keep your neck straight with your back, instead of collapsing forward and rounding the back and neck.

*At the computer, sit toward the edge of the seat with both or one foot under you and Zip Up. Sit on a stool when you can, or better yet a kneeling chair.

*Try to look up and down with your eyes, rather than bending your head over for any length of time.

*Be mindful about too much nodding.

Open Your Chest in Daily Activities

*Never cross arms in front of you, rather clasp hands behind your bottom, or rest hands on hips either facing up or down.

*Spread one or both arms out over top/back of couch when sitting. Do the same over tops of chairs next to you for instance seats in a theater or church pew.

*When writing or drawing, sit sideways to the table in order to open the shoulder of the arm you are writing with.

*For reading, sometimes sit sideways on the couch, legs curled, and hold the book on the back of the couch at eye level to keep from collapsing and looking down. Switch sides now and then and periodically stretch legs out.

*Driving – When it's safe, put your right arm behind the passenger seat, or hold on to the head rest.

*Do work tasks in front of you, and on a counter instead of bending over.

Lengthen Torso

*Lie on pillows from tail to base of skull, arms out to sides. Can use towel roll under neck too if desired.

*Lie back across bed with your head almost hanging over the edge, and arms spread out to sides on bed.

*Lie back on a large ball

*Periodically lean back in your chair with your hands interlaced behind your head with elbows out to the sides.

For Arms and Hands

*Foremost, **ALL** neck care hints are good for hands and arms, including the Zip It Up.

*Let your arms hang at your sides, perpendicular to the floor when typing, with elbows bent and wrists straight with your forearm. OR if your desk is high enough, slide your laptop away and rest your forearms on the table for a while.

*Do pectoral stretch gently as often as possible extending the stretch into forearms and wrists. (Use caution here if you have shoulder problems)

*Shake arms, hands and fingers out, up, down; feel the vibration up into your shoulders and neck.

*Softly stretch the insides of your hands everywhere – on counter tops, on the roof of your car while driving, against the head of the bed, on your thighs, and on your hips.

*Squeeze forearms between knees, as if ironing them out.

*Slap yourself all over to stimulate blood flow and flexibility. (Chi Gong)

*If you feel numbness or tingling of arms or hands, check to make sure your neck is in line with your spine.

*Stand up and with arms dangling loosely, twist your torso from side to side, letting your arms fling freely as if they were limp noodles.

*Use Pit Pillows

For your Low Back

*Stretch (gently) abdominal muscles by extending arms straight up overhead. No bending backward here.

*Stretch Quads gently, the front of your thighs. Bend knee, hold foot in hand behind you, or rest foot on a low stool or chair rung behind you.

*Change chairs now and then.

*If sitting on edge of chair, straighten each leg out alternately for a while.

*Soften your knees. By this I mean never lock them back, but rather let them be unconstrained as if you could go into a squat easily if you needed to. (Note – habitually locking your knees in standing will often lead to low back problems).

*Generally have feet parallel and hip width apart when standing / walking / sleeping.

*Shift weight side to side when standing, i.e. waiting in a line or on the job. This can be so subtle no one will notice.

*Do a gentle kick walk, with each step give a little kick before your foot hits the ground. Feel the vibration into your low back.

*Press trigger points in lateral Quads, the muscles on the outer edge of the front of your thigh.

*End of day – sit on the edge of the bed and lie back, arms overhead, to stretch out quads and abs. (may need a small pillow under your low back).

*Use a pillow between knees when side sleeping.

*Forget sit ups/crunches. Rather stretch torso with arms overhead and suck in (transverse) abdominals. Can be done lying down or standing.

For Knees

*Stretch your hamstrings. You can rest arms on the counter and go sway back, gently!

*While at computer, stretch a leg out to the side now and then.

*Movement is life! Instead of standing still while waiting in line, gently sway side to side.

Sleeping

*Sleeping on back with small support under neck is very good.

*If sleeping on side, put top arm on your side or leg to keep from collapsing forward. May use pillow in front of torso for arm rest.

*A thin pillow under your side can be very helpful, and in that case add thickness to your neck pillow.

*Try lying on your back, lace fingers and rest back of hands on forehead, elbows out to sides for a while.

<u>Change</u>

Remember our bodies are not meant to be static or to do repetitive motions for long periods.

Change periodically:

*chairs

*keyboard height

*mouse position

*shoes, if standing a lot

*pillows

These simple practices may be helpful in recovering numerous situations including:

-whiplash injuries

-disc problems

-sciatica

-upper cervical related headaches

-sinus pressure

-TMJ syndrome and bruxism

-other spinal related neuropathies

"Good posture and an attitude let you get away with anything."
— *Lorna Landvik, Angry Housewives Eating Bon Bons*

FINAL NOTE –

We are all different and carry a vast range of pressures at work and home, histories, accidents, and health challenges. Our work stations can vary from spacious and warm to cold and cramped. I know people who have worked at a desk for thirty years and only suffer occasional neck discomfort. I have seen clients who are debilitated from that same routine. Some of us are blessed with lifelong flexibility, sense of ease and positive attitude. Some of us are more easily overwhelmed and burdened with the deadlines, seemingly insurmountable tasks, and various co-workers we are given, leading to unbearable emotional tension and physical pain. Some of us are fortunate to find ourselves in a work environment that is uplifting and energizing, surrounded by friendly associates, while a common occurrence seems to be situations that are stressful at best. I hope that some of the information I've given is helpful to you in your particular circumstance, and my wish is that by finding balance in your body and at your work station, you will also find more balance in your way of being in the world.

Note – If you have pain that persists and is not resolved with the suggestions in this manual, you may have a more serious problem and I would recommend seeing a physical therapist or MD.

Suggested Reading:

East Meets West: An Integrative Approach to Managing Overuse Injury by Dr. Diane Gross, 2nd Edition. CreateSpace Publishing, 2014

Trager Mentastics; Movement as a Way to Agelessness by Milton Trager, M.D., and Cathy Hammond, Ph.D. Station Hill Press, Inc., 1995

To access the balance chair:

There doesn't seem to be an exact link that works, but if you google the following description you will see the kneeling chair –

'Office star ergonomically designed mahogany finished wood knee chair'

ABOUT THE AUTHOR:

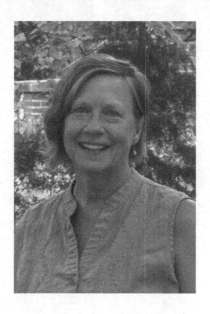

Bio

Betsy Oldenburg became certified in The Trager Approach®
in 1985, and graduated from the New Mexico Academy
of Advanced healing Arts in 1991. She has worked in a
chiropractic clinic, an orthopedic clinic, an acupuncture
center and has practiced at Integrative Therapies pain clinic
for twenty three years. Betsy has maintained a private
practice in Greensboro, NC for thirty years. She is a Trager
Practitioner and tutor, and a state certified massage therapist,
and has trained in numerous other modalities. Betsy teaches
classes designed to help restore bone mass called 'Bones for
Life®' based on the work of Dr. Moshe Feldenkrais. Her
latest passion is teaching a radical approach to ergonomics
she calls, "Look and Feel Great Despite Your Computer".

Printed in the United States
By Bookmasters